Blue Health &

Blue health refers to the positi͟ environments, such as oceans, lakes, and rivers, can have on our well-being. It's no secret that spending time by the water can bring a sense of calm and relaxation, helping to reduce stress and anxiety. The soothing sounds of waves crashing, the fresh sea breeze, and the sight of vast blue waters can all contribute to a feeling of peace and tranquility.

When it comes to connecting blue health with self-belief and confidence, the water's vastness can serve as a powerful metaphor. Just like the expansive blue ocean, our potential and capabilities are limitless. By immersing ourselves in the beauty of the water, we can be reminded of our own strength and resilience.

The sense of freedom and openness that comes with being near the water can inspire us to believe in ourselves and our abilities to overcome any challenges that come our way.

So, next time you're feeling uncertain or lacking in confidence, take a moment to soak in the blue health around you. Let the calming waters wash away any doubts and fears, and allow yourself to embrace the endless possibilities that lie ahead. Remember, just like the ocean, you are capable of great things

Natalia x

Be kind to yourself

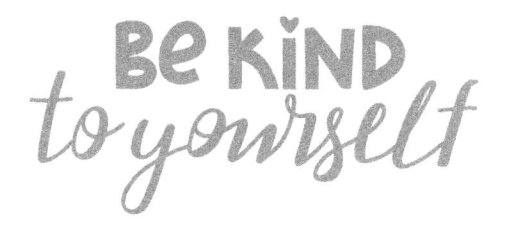

Daily Reminder

Always believe in yourself.
Even if you don't feel like you can
make it, keep pushing forward.
I promise you it will be worth it.
Make a plan and stick to it.
Your future self will be so grateful.

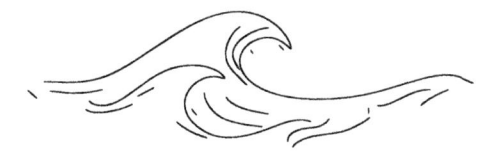

Self-Reflection Questions

Give one word answers only, and don't overthink it, write the first thought that comes to mind.

What is your first memory?	
What are you most proud of?	
What is something I have overcome?	
What was the best gift you've received?	
What's your favourite memory?	
Are you happy?	
What challenge are you currently facing?	
Do you feel content with life?	
What's your first thought waking up?	
Do you enjoy your life?	
Do you have goals?	

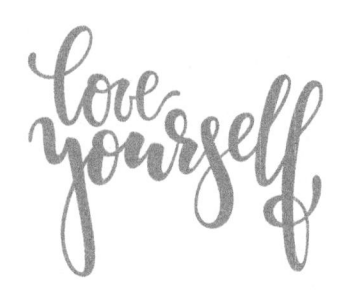

love yourself

20-DAY SELF-CARE *checklist*

DAY	TASK	DONE
01	Enjoy a healthy breakfast	☐
02	Take a 30-minute walk	☐
03	Meditate for 15 minutes	☐
04	Read a book for 30 minutes	☐
05	Write down 3 things you're grateful for	☐
06	Call a friend or family member	☐
07	Stretch for 15 minutes	☐
08	Drink 8 glasses of water	☐
09	Create a relaxing bedtime routine	☐
10	Listen to calming music	☐
11	Declutter your living space	☐
12	Cook a healthy meal	☐
13	Treat yourself to a relaxing bath or shower	☐
14	Set goals for the week ahead	☐
15	Practice deep breathing	☐
16	Write in a journal	☐
17	Spend 30 minutes in nature	☐
18	Listen to a podcast or inspirational talk	☐
19	Practice yoga or exercise	☐
20	Compliment yourself	☐

YOU'VE GOT THIS!

Is there anything in particular I'm struggling with?
Is there anything I can do to change this?

Do I feel that I live a balanced life with home, work, friendships, and relationships? If no, why not? Do I want to change this?

Do specific memories cheer me up? If so, do these relate to the location, the people I was with, music, or something else?

Do I believe in myself and know my self worth? If not, then why, what has triggered this?

Let my new journey begin,
time to journal...

SELF REFLECTIONS

THINGS I DO TO PROCESS MY FEELINGS

THINGS THAT KEEP ME BUSY

THINGS THAT MAKE ME FEEL CONFIDENT

FAVOURITE FEEL GOOD MUSIC

Do I have my favourite songs at home? Can I get them?

Why not start and end every day with listening to one of these tracks.

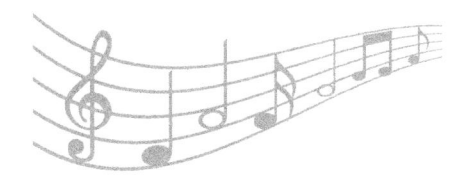

FAVOURITE HOBBIES

I AM
LIMITLESS

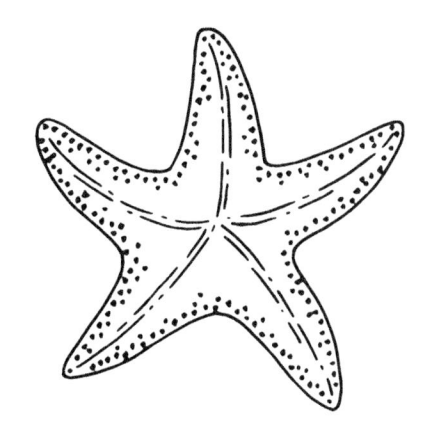

Dear journal...

DATE

WEEKLY REFLECTION

What did I achieve this week?

What did I learn this week?

What made me happy this week?

What was challenging this week?

Best moment of the week:

Intentions for next week:

Dear journal...

DATE

WEEKLY REFLECTION

What did I achieve this week?

What did I learn this week?

What made me happy this week?

What was challenging this week?

Best moment of the week:

Intentions for next week:

Dear journal...

DATE

WEEKLY REFLECTION

What did I achieve this week?

What did I learn this week?

What made me happy this week?

What was challenging this week?

Best moment of the week:

Intentions for next week:

Dear journal...

DATE

WEEKLY REFLECTION

What did I achieve this week?

What did I learn this week?

What made me happy this week?

What was challenging this week?

Best moment of the week:

Intentions for next week:

Dear journal...

DATE

WEEKLY REFLECTION

What did I achieve this week?

What did I learn this week?

What made me happy this week?

What was challenging this week?

Best moment of the week:

Intentions for next week:

Dear journal...

DATE

WEEKLY REFLECTION

What did I achieve this week?

What did I learn this week?

What made me happy this week?

What was challenging this week?

Best moment of the week:

Intentions for next week:

Dear journal...

DATE

WEEKLY REFLECTION

What did I achieve this week?

What did I learn this week?

What made me happy this week?

What was challenging this week?

Best moment of the week:

Intentions for next week:

I AM GOOD ENOUGH

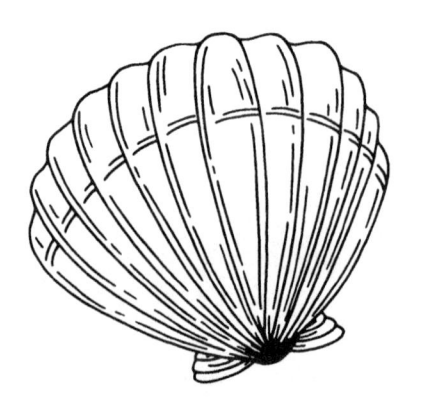

LIVING MY BEST LIFE

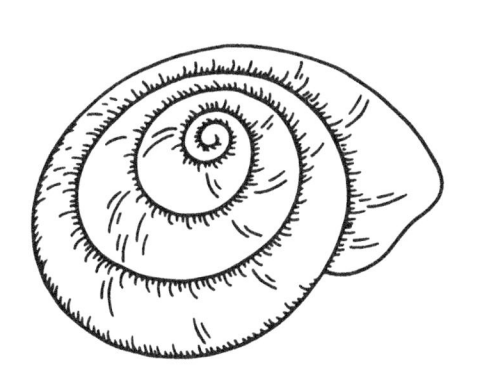

Dear journal...

DATE

WEEKLY REFLECTION

What did I achieve this week?

What did I learn this week?

What made me happy this week?

What was challenging this week?

Best moment of the week:

Intentions for next week:

Dear journal...

DATE

WEEKLY REFLECTION

What did I achieve this week?

What did I learn this week?

What made me happy this week?

What was challenging this week?

Best moment of the week:

Intentions for next week:

Dear journal...

DATE

WEEKLY REFLECTION

What did I achieve this week?

What did I learn this week?

What made me happy this week?

What was challenging this week?

Best moment of the week:

Intentions for next week:

Dear journal...

DATE

WEEKLY REFLECTION

What did I achieve this week?

What did I learn this week?

What made me happy this week?

What was challenging this week?

Best moment of the week:

Intentions for next week:

Dear journal...

DATE

WEEKLY REFLECTION

What did I achieve this week?

What did I learn this week?

What made me happy this week?

What was challenging this week?

Best moment of the week:

Intentions for next week:

Dear journal...

DATE

WEEKLY REFLECTION

What did I achieve this week?

What did I learn this week?

What made me happy this week?

What was challenging this week?

Best moment of the week:

Intentions for next week:

Dear journal...

DATE

WEEKLY REFLECTION

What did I achieve this week?

What did I learn this week?

What made me happy this week?

What was challenging this week?

Best moment of the week:

Intentions for next week:

Dear journal...

DATE

WEEKLY REFLECTION

What did I achieve this week?

What did I learn this week?

What made me happy this week?

What was challenging this week?

Best moment of the week:

Intentions for next week:

Dear journal...

DATE

WEEKLY REFLECTION

What did I achieve this week?

What did I learn this week?

What made me happy this week?

What was challenging this week?

Best moment of the week:

Intentions for next week:

Dear journal...

DATE

WEEKLY REFLECTION

What did I achieve this week?

What did I learn this week?

What made me happy this week?

What was challenging this week?

Best moment of the week:

Intentions for next week:

Dear journal...

DATE

WEEKLY REFLECTION

What did I achieve this week?

What did I learn this week?

What made me happy this week?

What was challenging this week?

Best moment of the week:

Intentions for next week:

Dear journal...

DATE

WEEKLY REFLECTION

What did I achieve this week?

What did I learn this week?

What made me happy this week?

What was challenging this week?

Best moment of the week:

Intentions for next week:

Dear journal...

DATE

WEEKLY REFLECTION

What did I achieve this week?

What did I learn this week?

What made me happy this week?

What was challenging this week?

Best moment of the week:

Intentions for next week:

Dear journal...

DATE

WEEKLY REFLECTION

What did I achieve this week?

What did I learn this week?

What made me happy this week?

What was challenging this week?

Best moment of the week:

Intentions for next week:

I WILL MAKE ME PROUD

I LEARN FROM MY MISTAKES

Dear journal...

DATE

WEEKLY REFLECTION

What did I achieve this week?

What did I learn this week?

What made me happy this week?

What was challenging this week?

Best moment of the week:

Intentions for next week:

Dear journal...

DATE

WEEKLY REFLECTION

What did I achieve this week?

What did I learn this week?

What made me happy this week?

What was challenging this week?

Best moment of the week:

Intentions for next week:

Dear journal...

DATE

WEEKLY REFLECTION

What did I achieve this week?

What did I learn this week?

What made me happy this week?

What was challenging this week?

Best moment of the week:

Intentions for next week:

Dear journal...

DATE

WEEKLY REFLECTION

What did I achieve this week?

What did I learn this week?

What made me happy this week?

What was challenging this week?

Best moment of the week:

Intentions for next week:

Dear journal...

DATE

WEEKLY REFLECTION

What did I achieve this week?

What did I learn this week?

What made me happy this week?

What was challenging this week?

Best moment of the week:

Intentions for next week:

Dear journal...

DATE

WEEKLY REFLECTION

What did I achieve this week?

What did I learn this week?

What made me happy this week?

What was challenging this week?

Best moment of the week:

Intentions for next week:

Dear journal...

DATE

WEEKLY REFLECTION

What did I achieve this week?

What did I learn this week?

What made me happy this week?

What was challenging this week?

Best moment of the week:

Intentions for next week:

Dear journal...

DATE

WEEKLY REFLECTION

What did I achieve this week?

What did I learn this week?

What made me happy this week?

What was challenging this week?

Best moment of the week:

Intentions for next week:

Dear journal...

DATE

WEEKLY REFLECTION

What did I achieve this week?

What did I learn this week?

What made me happy this week?

What was challenging this week?

Best moment of the week:

Intentions for next week:

Dear journal...

DATE

WEEKLY REFLECTION

What did I achieve this week?

What did I learn this week?

What made me happy this week?

What was challenging this week?

Best moment of the week:

Intentions for next week:

Dear journal...

DATE

WEEKLY REFLECTION

What did I achieve this week?

What did I learn this week?

What made me happy this week?

What was challenging this week?

Best moment of the week:

Intentions for next week:

Dear journal...

DATE

WEEKLY REFLECTION

What did I achieve this week?

What did I learn this week?

What made me happy this week?

What was challenging this week?

Best moment of the week:

Intentions for next week:

Dear journal...

DATE

WEEKLY REFLECTION

What did I achieve this week?

What did I learn this week?

What made me happy this week?

What was challenging this week?

Best moment of the week:

Intentions for next week:

Dear journal...

DATE

WEEKLY REFLECTION

What did I achieve this week?

What did I learn this week?

What made me happy this week?

What was challenging this week?

Best moment of the week:

Intentions for next week:

I AM IN CHARGE

ALWAYS
LOOKING
FORWARD

Dear journal...

DATE

WEEKLY REFLECTION

What did I achieve this week?

What did I learn this week?

What made me happy this week?

What was challenging this week?

Best moment of the week:

Intentions for next week:

Dear journal...

DATE

WEEKLY REFLECTION

What did I achieve this week?

What did I learn this week?

What made me happy this week?

What was challenging this week?

Best moment of the week:

Intentions for next week:

Dear journal...

DATE

WEEKLY REFLECTION

What did I achieve this week?

What did I learn this week?

What made me happy this week?

What was challenging this week?

Best moment of the week:

Intentions for next week:

Dear journal...

DATE

WEEKLY REFLECTION

What did I achieve this week?

What did I learn this week?

What made me happy this week?

What was challenging this week?

Best moment of the week:

Intentions for next week:

Dear journal...

DATE

WEEKLY REFLECTION

What did I achieve this week?

What did I learn this week?

What made me happy this week?

What was challenging this week?

Best moment of the week:

Intentions for next week:

Dear journal...

DATE

WEEKLY REFLECTION

What did I achieve this week?

What did I learn this week?

What made me happy this week?

What was challenging this week?

Best moment of the week:

Intentions for next week:

Dear journal...

DATE

WEEKLY REFLECTION

What did I achieve this week?

What did I learn this week?

What made me happy this week?

What was challenging this week?

Best moment of the week:

Intentions for next week:

Dear journal...

DATE

WEEKLY REFLECTION

What did I achieve this week?

What did I learn this week?

What made me happy this week?

What was challenging this week?

Best moment of the week:

Intentions for next week:

Dear journal...

DATE

WEEKLY REFLECTION

What did I achieve this week?

What did I learn this week?

What made me happy this week?

What was challenging this week?

Best moment of the week:

Intentions for next week:

Dear journal...

DATE

WEEKLY REFLECTION

What did I achieve this week?

What did I learn this week?

What made me happy this week?

What was challenging this week?

Best moment of the week:

Intentions for next week:

Dear journal...

DATE

WEEKLY REFLECTION

What did I achieve this week?

What did I learn this week?

What made me happy this week?

What was challenging this week?

Best moment of the week:

Intentions for next week:

Dear journal...

DATE

WEEKLY REFLECTION

What did I achieve this week?

What did I learn this week?

What made me happy this week?

What was challenging this week?

Best moment of the week:

Intentions for next week:

Dear journal...

DATE

WEEKLY REFLECTION

What did I achieve this week?

What did I learn this week?

What made me happy this week?

What was challenging this week?

Best moment of the week:

Intentions for next week:

Dear journal...

DATE

WEEKLY REFLECTION

What did I achieve this week?

What did I learn this week?

What made me happy this week?

What was challenging this week?

Best moment of the week:

Intentions for next week:

STRONG
&
BEAUTIFUL

I CAN REACH MY GOALS

Dear journal...

DATE

WEEKLY REFLECTION

What did I achieve this week?

What did I learn this week?

What made me happy this week?

What was challenging this week?

Best moment of the week:

Intentions for next week:

Dear journal...

DATE

WEEKLY REFLECTION

What did I achieve this week?

What did I learn this week?

What made me happy this week?

What was challenging this week?

Best moment of the week:

Intentions for next week:

Dear journal...

DATE

WEEKLY REFLECTION

What did I achieve this week?

What did I learn this week?

What made me happy this week?

What was challenging this week?

Best moment of the week:

Intentions for next week:

TIME IS MY BIGGEST ASSET

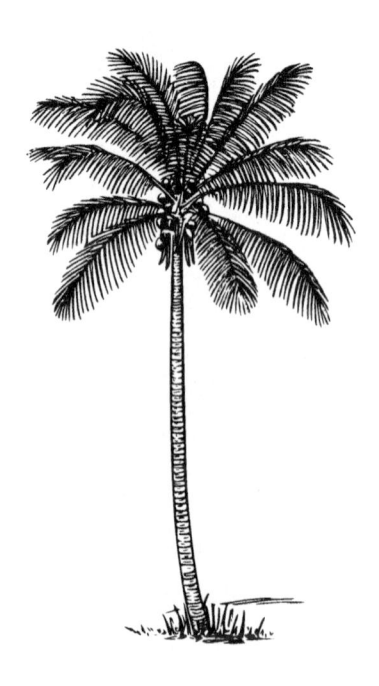

NOTES

notes

DATE / /

notes

DATE / /

notes

DATE   /   /

notes

DATE   /   /

notes   DATE   /   /

notes

DATE   /   /

notes

DATE   /   /

notes

DATE   /   /

notes DATE   /   /

notes

DATE   /   /

notes

DATE   /   /

notes

DATE   /   /

You Are Enough